A Beginner Guide to Prepare Your Own Keto Chaffle

50 Fast, Simple, and Tasty Recipes to Boost Your Metabolism

Catherine Willis

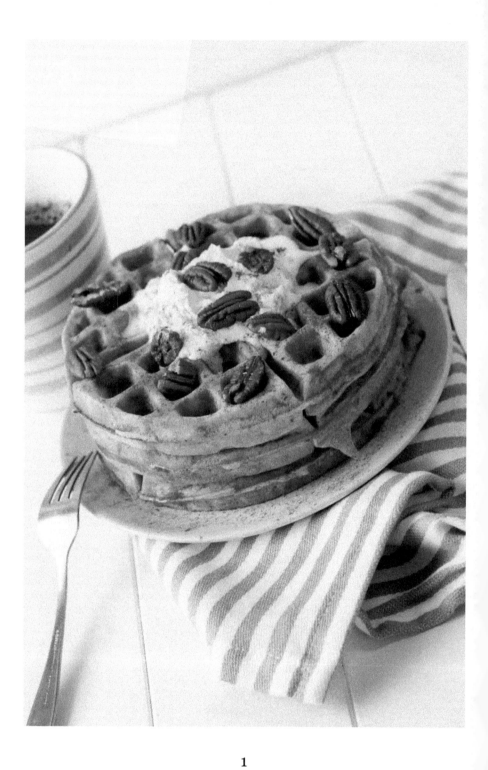

sources. Please consult a licensed professional before attempting any techniques outlined in this book.

By reading this document, the reader agrees that under no circumstances is the author responsible for any losses, direct or indirect, which are incurred as a result of the use of information contained within this document, including, but not limited to, — errors, omissions, or inaccuracies.

Table of Contents

Crispy Bagel Chaffles

Preparation time : 5 minutes

Cooking Time : 30 Minutes

Servings : 2

INGREDIENTS :

   2 eggs

   ½ cup parmesan cheese

   1 tsp bagel seasoning

   ½ cup mozzarella cheese

   2 teaspoons almond flour

DIRECTIONS :

1. Turn on the waffle maker to heat and oil it with cooking spray.
2. Evenly sprinkle half of the cheeses on a grill and let them melt. Then toast for 30 seconds and leave them waiting for the batter.
3. Whisk eggs, other half of cheeses, almond flour, and bagel seasoning in a small bowl.
4. Pour batter into the waffle maker. Cook for minutes.
5. Let cool for 2-3 minutes before serving.

NUTRITION :Carbs: g;Fat: 20 g;Protein: 21 g;Calories: 287

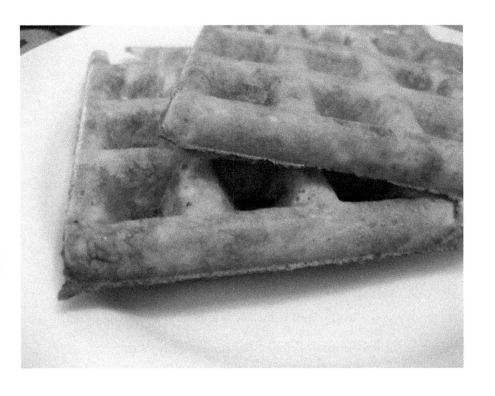

Sausage & Veggies Chaffles

Preparation time : 10 minutes

Cooking Time : 20 Minutes

Servings : 2

INGREDIENTS :

    1/3 cup unsweetened almond milk

    4 medium organic eggs

    2 tablespoons gluten-free breakfast sausage, cut into slices

    2 tablespoons broccoli florets, chopped

    2 tablespoons bell peppers, seeded and chopped

    2 tablespoons Mozzarella cheese, shredded

DIRECTIONS :

1. Preheat a waffle iron and then grease it.
2. In a medium bowl, place the almond milk and eggs and beat well.
3. Place the remaining **INGREDIENTS** and stir to combine well.
4. Place ¼ of the mixture into preheated waffle iron and cook for about 5 minutes or until golden brown.
5. Repeat with the remaining mixture.
6. Serve warm.

NUTRITION :

Calories: 132Net Carb: 1.2gFat: 9.2gSaturated Fat: 3.5gCarbohydrates: 1.4gDietary Fiber: 0.2g Sugar: 0.5gProtein: 11.1g

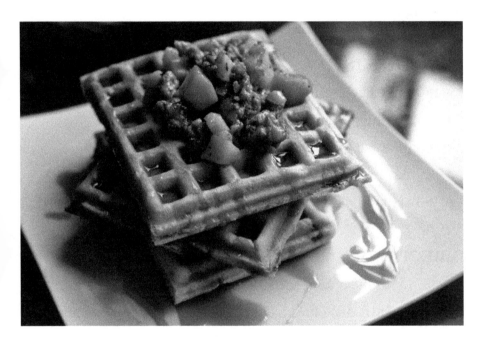

Broccoli & Almond Flour Waffles

Preparation time : 6 minutes

Cooking Time : 8 Minutes

Servings : 2

INGREDIENTS :
- 1 organic egg, beaten
- ½ cup Cheddar cheese, shredded
- ¼ cup fresh broccoli, chopped
- 1 tablespoon almond flour
- ¼ teaspoon garlic powder

DIRECTIONS :
1. Preheat a mini waffle iron and then grease it.
2. Introduce to a medium bowl, all ingredients and mix until well combined.
3. Put a portion of the mixture into preheated waffle iron and cook for about 4 minutes or until golden brown.
4. Repeat with the remaining mixture.
5. Serve warm.

NUTRITION :

Calories: 173Net Carb: 1.5gFat: 13.5gSaturated Fat: 8gCarbohydrates: 2.2gDietary Fiber: 0.7g Sugar: 0.7gProtein: 10.2g

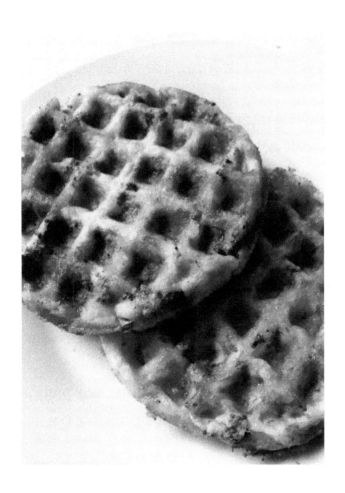

Bacon & Serrano Pepper Chaffles

Preparation time : 6 minutes

Cooking Time : 10 Minutes

Servings : 2

INGREDIENTS :

    1 organic egg, beaten

    ½ cup Swiss/Gruyere cheese blend, shredded

    2 tablespoons cooked bacon slices, chopped

    1 tablespoon Serrano pepper, chopped

DIRECTIONS :

1. Preheat a mini waffle iron and then grease it.
2. Introduce to a medium bowl, all ingredients and mix until well combined.
3. Put a portion of the mixture into preheated waffle iron and cook for about 5 minutes or until golden brown.
4. Repeat with the remaining mixture.
5. Meanwhile, for dip: in a bowl, mix the cream and stevia.
6. Serve warm.

NUTRITION : Calories: 141Net Carb: 1.Fat: 10.2gSaturated Fat: 5.7gCarbohydrates: 1.8gDietary Fiber: 0.1g Sugar: 0.7gProtein: 10.5g

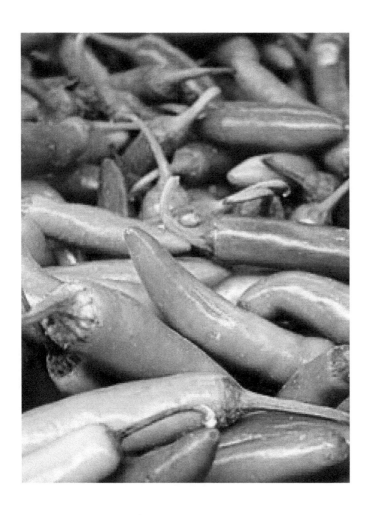

Garlic Powder Chaffles

Preparation time : 6 minutes

Cooking Time : 8 Minutes

Servings : 2

INGREDIENTS :

    1 organic egg, beaten

    ½ cup Monterey Jack cheese, shredded

    1 teaspoon coconut flour

    Pinch of garlic powder

DIRECTIONS :

1. Preheat a mini waffle iron and then grease it.
2. Add all ingredients in a bowl and combine until well mixed.
3. Put a portion of the mixture in the preheated waffle iron and cook until golden brown, or around 4 minutes.
4. Repeat with the mixture that remains.
5. Serve it hot.

NUTRITION : Calories: 147Net Carb: 1.Fat: 11.3gSaturated Fat: 6.8gCarbohydrates: 2.1gDietary Fiber: 0.5g Sugar: 0.2gProtein: 9g

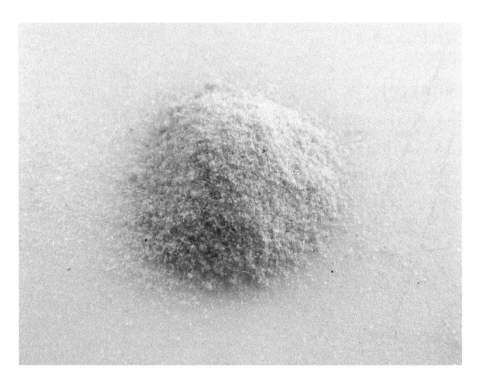

Aioli Chicken Waffle Sandwich

Preparation time : 5 minutes

Cooking Time : 6 Minutes

Servings : 2

INGREDIENTS :

    ¼ cup shredded rotisserie chicken

    2 Tbsp Kewpie mayo

    ½ tsp lemon juice

    1 grated garlic clove

    ¼ green onion, chopped

    1 egg

    ½ cup shredded mozzarella cheese

DIRECTIONS :

1. Mix lemon juice and mayo in a small bowl.
2. Turn on the waffle maker to heat and oil it with cooking spray.
3. Beat egg in a small bowl.
4. Place ⅛ cup of cheese on the waffle maker, then spread half of the egg mixture over it and top with ⅛ cup of cheese. Close and cook for 3-minutes.
5. Repeat for remaining batter.

6. Place chicken on chaffles and top with sauce. Sprinkle with chopped green onion

NUTRITION :Carbs: 3 g;Fat: 42 g;Protein: 34 g;Calories: 545

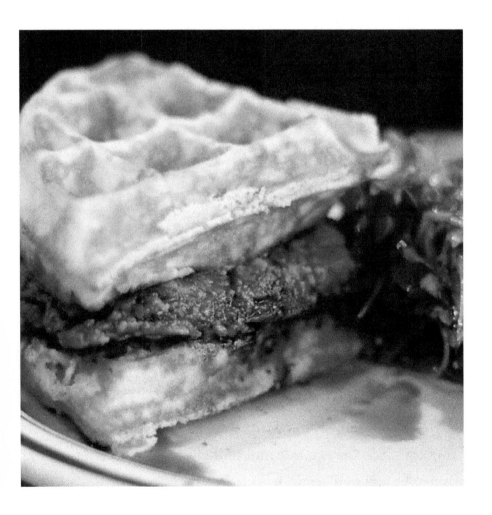

Sage & Coconut Milk Chaffles

Servings : 6

Cooking Time : 24 Minutes

INGREDIENTS :

    ¾ cup coconut flour, sifted

    1½ teaspoons organic baking powder

    ½ teaspoon dried ground sage

    1/8 teaspoon garlic powder

    1/8 teaspoon salt

    1 organic egg

    1 cup unsweetened coconut milk

    ¼ cup water

    1½ tablespoons coconut oil, melted

    ½ cup cheddar cheese, shredded

DIRECTIONS :

1. Preheat a waffle iron and then grease it.
2. In a bowl, add the flour, baking powder, sage, garlic powder, salt, and mix well.
3. Add the egg, coconut milk, water and coconut oil and mix until a stiff mixture forms.
4. Add the cheese and gently stir to combine.

19

5. Divide the mixture into 6 portions.

6. Place 1 portion of the mixture into preheated waffle iron and cook for about 4 minutes or until golden brown.

7. Repeat with the remaining mixture.

8. Serve warm.

NUTRITION : Calories: 147Net Carb: 2.2gFat: 13gSaturated Fat: 10.7gCarbohydrates: 2.Dietary Fiber: 0.7g Sugar: 1.3gProtein: 4 g

Chaffle Burger

Preparation time : 5 minutes

Cooking Time : 10 Minutes

Servings : 2

INGREDIENTS :

    For the burger:

    ⅓-pound ground beef

    ½ tsp garlic salt

    2 slices American cheese

    For the chaffles:

    1 large egg

    ½ cup shredded mozzarella

    ¼ tsp garlic salt

    For the sauce:

    2 tsp mayonnaise

    1 tsp ketchup

    1 tsp dill pickle relish

    splash vinegar, to taste

    For the toppings:

    2 Tbsp shredded lettuce

    3-4 dill pickles

    2 tsp onion, minced

DIRECTIONS :

1. Heat a griddle over medium-high heat.
2. Divide ground beef into balls and place on the grill, 6 inches apart. Cook for 1 minute.
3. Use a small plate to flatten beef. Sprinkle it with garlic salt.
4. Cook for 2-3, until halfway cooked through. Flip and sprinkle with garlic salt.
5. Cook for 2-3 minutes, or until cooked completely.
6. Place cheese slices over each patty and stack patties. Set aside on a plate. Cover with foil.
7. Turn on the waffle maker to heat and oil it with cooking spray.
8. Whisk egg, cheese, and garlic salt until well combined.
9. Add half of the egg mixture to the waffle maker and cook for 2-3 minutes.
10. Set aside and repeat with remaining batter.
11. Whisk all sauce ingredients in a bowl.
12. Top one chaffle with the stacked burger patties, shredded lettuce, pickles, and onions.
13. Spread sauce over the other chaffle and place sauce side down over the sandwich.
14. Eat immediately.

NUTRITION :Carbs: 8 g;Fat: 56 g;Protein: 65 g;Calories: 831

Vegan Chaffle

Preparation time : 5 minutes

Cooking Time : 25 Minutes

INGREDIENTS :

    1 Tbsp flaxseed meal

    2 ½ Tbsp water

    ¼ cup low carb vegan cheese

    2 Tbsp coconut flour

    1 Tbsp low carb vegan cream cheese, softened

    Pinch of salt

DIRECTIONS :

1. Turn on the waffle maker to heat and oil it with cooking spray.
2. Mix flaxseed and water in a bowl. Leave for 5 minutes, until thickened and gooey.
3. Whisk remaining **INGREDIENTS** for chaffle.
4. Pour one half of the batter into the center of the waffle maker. Close and cook for 3-5 minutes.
5. Remove chaffle and serve.

NUTRITION :Carbs: 33 g;Fat: 25 g;Protein: 25 g;Calories: 450

Lemony Fresh Herbs Chaffles

Servings : 6

Cooking Time : 24 Minutes

INGREDIENTS :

½ cup ground flaxseed

2 organic eggs

½ cup goat cheddar cheese, grated

2-4 tablespoons plain Greek yogurt

1 tablespoon avocado oil

½ teaspoon baking soda

1 teaspoon fresh lemon juice

2 tablespoons fresh chives, minced

1 tablespoon fresh basil, minced

½ tablespoon fresh mint, minced

¼ tablespoon fresh thyme, minced

¼ tablespoon fresh oregano, minced

Salt

freshly ground black pepper

DIRECTIONS :

1. Preheat a waffle iron and then grease it.
2. Introduce to a medium bowl, all ingredients and mix until well combined.

3. Divide the mixture into 6 portions.

4. Place 1 portion of the mixture into preheated waffle iron and cook for about minutes or until golden brown.

5. Repeat with the remaining mixture.

6. Serve warm.

NUTRITION : Calories: 11et Carb: 0.9gFat: 7.9gSaturated Fat: 3gCarbohydrates: 3.7gDietary Fiber: 2.8g Sugar: 0.7gProtein: 6.4 g

Italian Seasoning Chaffles

Preparation time : 6 minutes

Cooking Time : 8 Minutes

Servings : 2

INGREDIENTS :

    ½ cup Mozzarella cheese, shredded

    1 tablespoon Parmesan cheese, shredded

    1 organic egg

    ¾ teaspoon coconut flour

    ¼ teaspoon organic baking powder

    1/8 teaspoon Italian seasoning

    Pinch of salt

DIRECTIONS :

1. Preheat a mini waffle iron and then grease it.
2. Introduce to a medium bowl, all ingredients and mix until well combined.
3. Put a portion of the mixture in the preheated waffle iron and cook until golden brown, or around 4 minutes.
4. Repeat with the mixture that remains.
5. Serve it hot

NUTRITION : Calories: 8et Carb: 1.9gFat: 5gSaturated Fat: 2.6gCarbohydrates: 3.8gDietary Fiber: 1.9g Sugar: 0.6gProtein: 6.5g

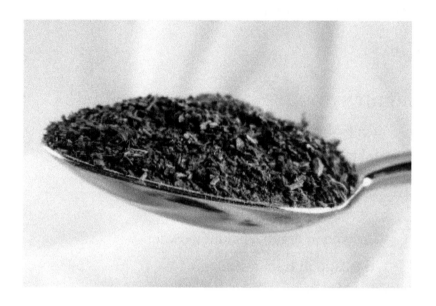

Basil Chaffles

Preparation time : 10 minutes

Cooking Time : 16 Minutes

Servings : 2

INGREDIENTS :

2 organic eggs, beaten

½ cup Mozzarella cheese, shredded

1 tablespoon Parmesan cheese, grated

1 teaspoon dried basil, crushed

Pinch of salt

DIRECTIONS :

1. Preheat a mini waffle iron and then grease it.
2. Introduce to a medium bowl, all ingredients and mix until well combined.
3. Place 1/of the mixture into preheated waffle iron and cook for about 3-4 minutes or until golden brown.
4. Repeat with the remaining mixture.
5. Serve warm.

NUTRITION : Calories: Net Carb: 0.4gFat: 4.2gSaturated Fat: 1.6gCarbohydrates: 0.4gDietary Fiber: 0g Sugar: 0.2gProtein: 5.7g

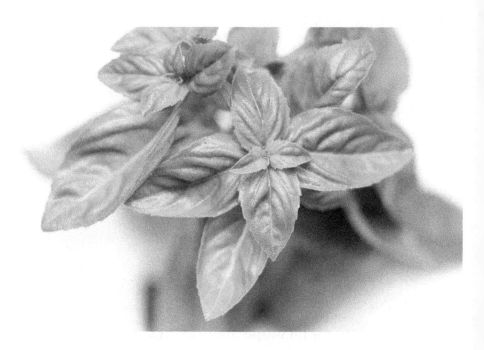

Bacon Chaffles

Preparation time : 6 minutes

Cooking Time : 5 Minutes

Servings : 2

INGREDIENTS :

    2 eggs

    ½ cup cheddar cheese

    ½ cup mozzarella cheese

    ¼ tsp baking powder

    ½ Tbsp almond flour

    1 Tbsp butter, for waffle maker

    For the filling:

    ¼ cup bacon, chopped

    2 Tbsp green onions, chopped

DIRECTIONS :

1. Turn on the waffle maker to heat and oil it with cooking spray.

2. Add eggs, mozzarella, cheddar, almond flour, and baking powder to a blender and pulse 10 times, so cheese is still chunky.

3. Add bacon and green onions. Pulse 2-times to combine.

4. Introduce a portion of the batter to the waffle maker and cook for 3 minutes, until golden brown.
5. Repeat with remaining batter.
6. Add your toppings and serve hot.

NUTRITION :Carbs: 3 g;Fat: 38 g;Protein: 23 g;Calories: 446

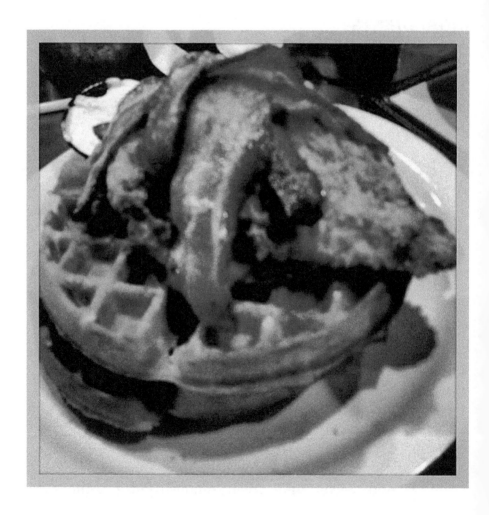

Sausage Chaffles

Preparation time : 5 minutes

Cooking Time : 1 Hour

Servings : 2

INGREDIENTS :

    1 pound gluten-free bulk Italian sausage, crumbled

    1 organic egg, beaten

    1 cup sharp Cheddar cheese, shredded

    ¼ cup Parmesan cheese, grated

    1 cup almond flour

    2 teaspoons organic baking powder

DIRECTIONS :

1. Preheat a mini waffle iron and then grease it.
2. Introduce to a medium bowl, all ingredients and mix until well combined.
3. Place about 3 tablespoons of the mixture into preheated waffle iron and cook for about 3 minutes or until golden brown.
4. Carefully, flip the chaffle and cook for about 2 minutes or until golden brown.
5. Repeat with the remaining mixture.
6. Serve warm.

NUTRITION : Calories: 238Net Carb: 1.2gFat: 19.6gSaturated Fat: 6.1gCarbohydrates: 2.2gDietary Fiber: 1g Sugar: 0.4gProtein: 10.8g

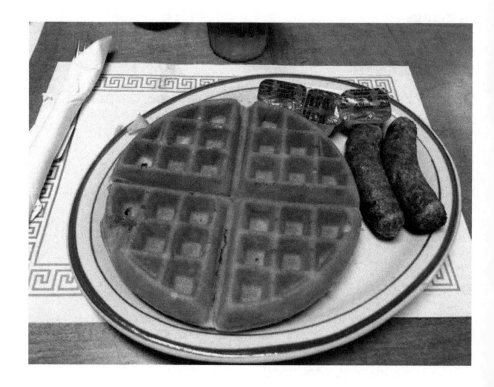

Scallion Cream Cheese Chaffle

Preparation time : 6 minutes

Cooking Time : 20 Minutes

Servings : 2

INGREDIENTS :

    1 large egg

    ½ cup of shredded mozzarella

    2 Tbsp cream cheese

    1 Tbsp everything bagel seasoning

    1-2 sliced scallions

DIRECTIONS :

1. Turn on the waffle maker to heat and oil it with cooking spray.
2. Beat egg in a small bowl.
3. Add in ½ cup mozzarella.
4. Introduce half of the mixture into the waffle maker and cook for 3-minutes.
5. Remove shuffle and repeat with remaining mixture.
6. Let them cool, then cover each chaffle with cream cheese, sprinkle with seasoning and scallions.

NUTRITION :Carbs: 8 g;Fat: 11 g;Protein: 5 g;Calories: 168

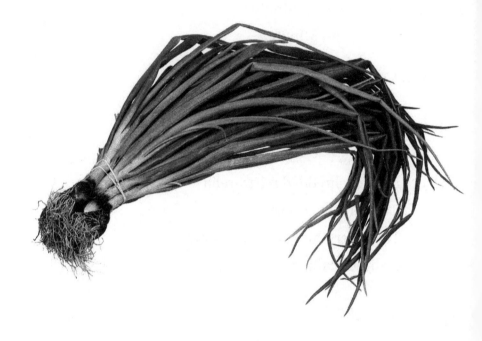

Broccoli Chaffles

Preparation time : 6 minutes

Cooking Time : 8 Minutes

Servings : 2

INGREDIENTS :

1/3 cup raw broccoli, chopped finely

¼ cup Cheddar cheese, shredded

1 organic egg

½ teaspoons garlic powder

½ teaspoons dried onion, minced

Salt

freshly ground black pepper

DIRECTIONS :

1. Preheat a mini waffle iron and then grease it.
2. Introduce to a medium bowl, all ingredients and mix until well combined.
3. Place ¼ of the mixture into preheated waffle iron and cook for about 4 minutes or until golden brown.
4. Repeat with the remaining mixture.
5. Serve warm.

NUTRITION : Calories: 9et Carb: 1.5gFat: 6.9gSaturated Fat: 3.7gCarbohydrates: 2gDietary Fiber: 0.5g Sugar: 0.7gProtein: 6.8g

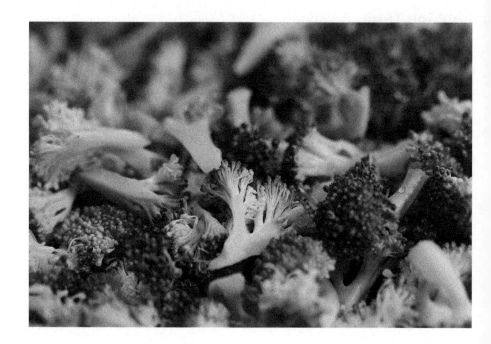

Chicken Taco Chaffles

Preparation time : 6 minutes

Cooking Time : 8 Minutes

Servings : 2

INGREDIENTS :

    1/3 cup cooked grass-fed chicken, chopped

    1 organic egg

    1/3 cup Monterey Jack cheese, shredded

    ¼ teaspoon taco seasoning

DIRECTIONS :

1. Preheat a mini waffle iron and then grease it.
2. Introduce to a medium bowl, all ingredients and mix until well combined.
3. Put a portion of the mixture in the preheated waffle iron and cook until golden brown, or around 4 minutes.
4. Repeat with the mixture that remains.
5. Serve it hot.

NUTRITION : Calories: 141Net Carb: 1.1gFat: 8.9gSaturated Fat: 4.9gCarbohydrates: 1.1gDietary Fiber: 0g Sugar: 0.2gProtein: 13.5g

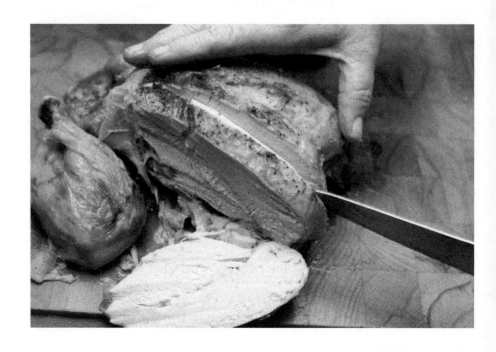

Bacon & 3-cheese Chaffles

Preparation time : 10 minutes

Cooking Time : 8 Minutes

Servings : 2

INGREDIENTS :

    3 large organic eggs

    ½ cup Swiss cheese, grated

    1/3 cup Parmesan cheese, grated

    1/4 cup cream cheese, softened

    4 tablespoons almond flour

    1 tablespoon coconut flour

    ½ teaspoon onion powder

    ½ teaspoon garlic powder

    ½ teaspoon dried basil, crushed

    ½ teaspoon dried oregano, crushed

    ½ teaspoon organic baking powder

    Salt

    freshly ground black pepper

    4 cooked bacon slices, cut in half

DIRECTIONS :

1.   Preheat a waffle iron and then grease it.

2. Introduce to a medium bowl, all ingredients without the bacon and mix until well combined.
3. Place ¼ of the mixture into preheated waffle iron.
4. Arrange 2 halved bacon slices over mixture and cook for about 2 minutes or until golden brown.
5. Repeat with the remaining mixture and bacon slices.
6. Serve warm.

NUTRITION : Calories: 259Net Carb: 3.2gFat: 20.1gSaturated Fat: 8.Carbohydrates: 4.8gDietary Fiber: 1.6g Sugar: 1gProtein: 13.9g

Spinach Chaffles

Preparation time : 10 minutes

Cooking Time : 20 Minutes

Servings : 2

INGREDIENTS :

    1 large organic egg, beaten

    1 cup ricotta cheese, crumbled

    ½ cup Mozzarella cheese, shredded

    ¼ cup Parmesan cheese, grated

    4 ounces frozen spinach, thawed and squeezed

    1 garlic clove, minced

    Salt

    freshly ground black pepper

DIRECTIONS :

1. Preheat a mini waffle iron and then grease it.
2. Introduce to a medium bowl, all ingredients and mix until well combined.
3. Place ¼ of the mixture into preheated waffle iron and cook for about 4-5 minutes or until golden brown.
4. Repeat with the remaining mixture.
5. Serve warm.

NUTRITION : Calories: 139Net Carb: 4.3gFat: 8.1gSaturated Fat: 4gCarbohydrates: 4.7gDietary Fiber: 0.4g Sugar: 0.4gProtein: 12.5g

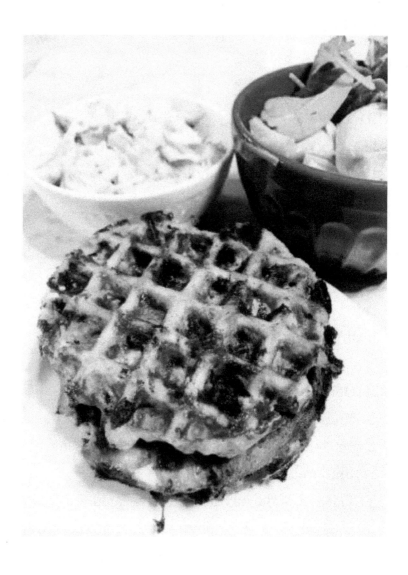

Ground Beef Chaffles

Preparation time : 10 minutes

Cooking Time : 20 Minutes

Servings : 2

INGREDIENTS :

 ½ cup cooked grass-fed ground beef

 3 cooked bacon slices, chopped

 2 organic eggs

 ½ cup Cheddar cheese, shredded

 ½ cup Mozzarella cheese, shredded

 2 teaspoons steak seasoning

DIRECTIONS :

1. Preheat a mini waffle iron and then grease it.
2. Introduce to a medium bowl, all ingredients and mix until well combined.
3. Place ¼ of the mixture into preheated waffle iron and cook for about 4-5 minutes or until golden brown.
4. Repeat with the remaining mixture.
5. Serve warm.

NUTRITION : Calories: 214Net Carb: 0.gFat: 12gSaturated Fat: 5.7gCarbohydrates: 0.5gDietary Fiber: g Sugar: 0.2gProtein: 2.1g

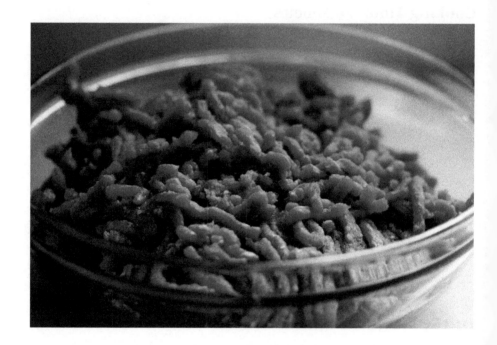

Chicken & Bacon Chaffles

Preparation time : 6 minutes

Cooking Time : 8 Minutes

Servings : 2

INGREDIENTS :

    1 organic egg, beaten

    1/3 cup grass-fed cooked chicken, chopped

    1 cooked bacon slice, crumbled

    1/3 cup Pepper Jack cheese, shredded

    1 teaspoon powdered ranch dressing

DIRECTIONS :

1. Preheat a mini waffle iron and then grease it.
2. Introduce to a medium bowl, all ingredients and mix until well combined
3. Put a portion of the mixture in the preheated waffle iron and cook until golden brown, or around 4 minutes.
4. Repeat with the mixture that remains.
5. Serve it hot.

NUTRITION : Calories: 145Net Carb: 0.9gFat: 9.4gSaturated Fat: 4.Carbohydrates: 1gDietary Fiber: 0.1g Sugar: 0.2gProtein: 14.3g

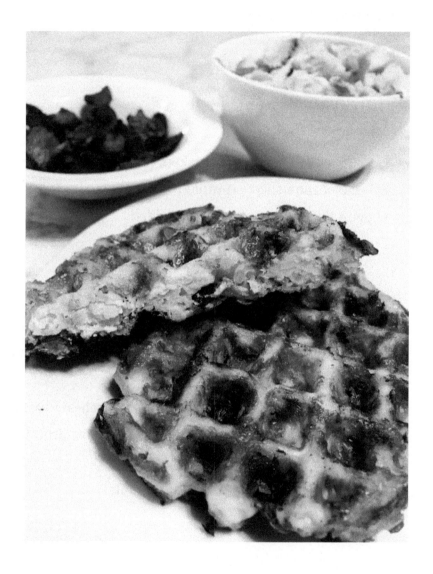

Belgium Waffles

Preparation time : 5 minutes

Cooking Time : 6 Minutes

Servings : 2

INGREDIENTS :

2 eggs

1 cup Reduced-fat Cheddar cheese, shredded

DIRECTIONS :

1. Turn on the waffle maker to heat and oil it with cooking spray.
2. Whisk eggs in a bowl, add cheese. Stir until well-combined.
3. Pour mixture into the waffle maker and cook for 6 minutes until done.
4. Let it cool a little until crisp before serving.

NUTRITION :Carbs: 2 g;Fat: 33 g;Protein: 44 g;Calories: 460

Salmon Chaffles

Preparation time : 6 minutes

Cooking Time : 10 Minutes

Servings : 2

INGREDIENTS :

1 large egg

½ cup shredded mozzarella

1 Tbsp cream cheese

2 slices salmon

1 Tbsp everything bagel seasoning

DIRECTIONS :

1. Turn on the waffle maker to heat and oil it with cooking spray.

2. Beat egg in a bowl, then add ½ cup mozzarella.

3. Introduce half of the mixture into the waffle maker and cook for 4 minutes.

4. Remove and repeat with remaining mixture.

5. Let chaffles cool, then spread cream cheese, sprinkle with seasoning, and top with salmon.

NUTRITION :Carbs: 3 g;Fat: 10 g;Protein: 5 g;Calories: 201

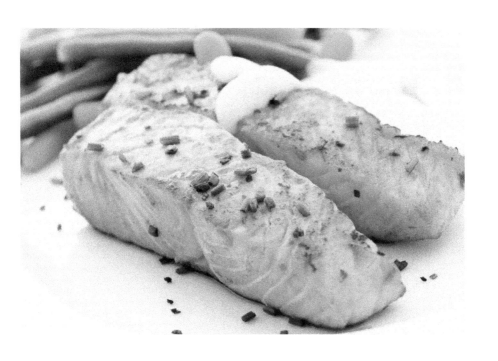

Chaffle Katsu Sandwich

Preparation time : 10 minutes

Cooking Time : 00 Minutes

Servings : 2

INGREDIENTS :

For the chicken:

¼ lb boneless and skinless chicken thigh

⅛ tsp salt

⅛ tsp black pepper

½ cup almond flour

1 egg

3 oz unflavored pork rinds

2 cup vegetable oil for deep frying

For the brine:

2 cup of water

1 Tbsp salt

For the sauce:

2 Tbsp sugar-free ketchup

1½ Tbsp Worcestershire Sauce

1 Tbsp oyster sauce

1 tsp swerve/monk fruit

For the chaffle:

2 egg

1 cup shredded mozzarella cheese

DIRECTIONS :

1. Add brine **INGREDIENTS** in a large mixing bowl.
2. Add chicken and brine for 1 hour.
3. Pat chicken dry with a paper towel. Sprinkle with salt and pepper. Set aside.
4. Mix ketchup, oyster sauce, Worcestershire sauce, and swerve in a small mixing bowl.
5. Pulse pork rinds in a food processor, making fine crumbs.
6. Fill one bowl with flour, a second bowl with beaten eggs, and a third with crushed pork rinds.
7. Dip and coat each thigh in: flour, eggs, crushed pork rinds. Transfer on holding a plate.
8. Add oil to cover ½ inch of frying pan. Heat to 375°F.
9. When hot, lower heat and add chicken.
10. Transfer to a drying rack.
11. Turn on the waffle maker to heat and oil it with cooking spray.
12. Beat egg in a small bowl.
13. Place ⅛ cup of cheese on the waffle maker, then add¼ of the egg mixture and top with ⅛ cup of cheese.
14. Cook for 3-4 minutes.

15. Repeat for remaining batter.

16. Top chaffles with chicken katsu, 1 Tbsp sauce, and another piece of chaffle.

NUTRITION :Carbs: 12 g;Fat: 1 g;Protein: 2 g;Calories: 57

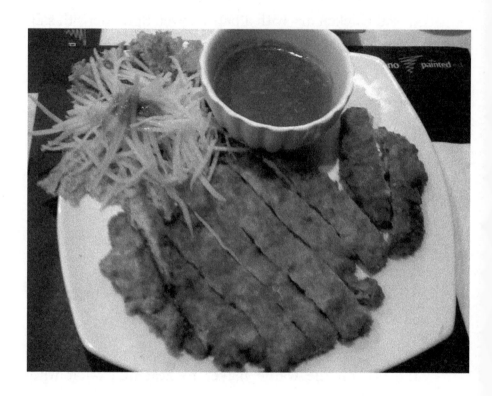

Pork Rind Chaffles

Preparation time : 6 minutes

Cooking Time : 10 Minutes

Servings : 2

INGREDIENTS :

      1 organic egg, beaten

      ½ cup ground pork rinds

      1/3 cup Mozzarella cheese, shredded

      Pinch of salt

DIRECTIONS :

1. Preheat a mini waffle iron and then grease it.
2. Introduce to a medium bowl, all ingredients and mix until well combined.
3. 3. Put a portion of the mixture in the preheated waffle iron and cook until golden brown, or around 5 minutes.
4. Repeat with the remaining mixture.
5. Serve warm.

NUTRITION : Calories: 91Net Carb: 0.3gFat: 5.9gSaturated Fat: 2.3gCarbohydrates: 0.3gDietary Fiber: 0g Sugar: 0.2gProtein: 9.2g

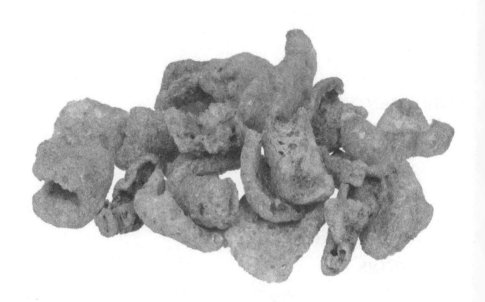

Chaffle Bruschetta

Preparation time : 5 minutes

Cooking Time : 5 Minutes

Servings : 2

INGREDIENTS :

    ½ cup shredded mozzarella cheese

    1 whole egg beaten

    ¼ cup grated Parmesan cheese

    1 tsp Italian Seasoning

    ¼ tsp garlic powder

    For the toppings:

    3-4 cherry tomatoes, chopped

    1 tsp fresh basil, chopped

    Splash of olive oil

    Pinch of salt

DIRECTIONS :

1. Turn on the waffle maker to heat and oil it with cooking spray.
2. Whisk all chaffle **INGREDIENTS** , except mozzarella, in a bowl.
3. Add in cheese and mix.

4. Add batter to the waffle maker and cook for 5 minutes.

5. Mix tomatoes, basil, olive oil, and salt. Serve over the top of chaffles.

NUTRITION :Carbs: 2 g;Fat: 24 g;Protein: 34 g;Calories: 352

Cheddar Protein Chaffles

Servings : 8

Cooking Time : 40 Minutes

INGREDIENTS :

  ½ cup golden flax seeds meal

  ½ cup almond flour

  2 tablespoons unsweetened whey protein powder

  1 teaspoon organic baking powder

  Sal

  freshly ground black pepper

  ¾ cup Cheddar cheese, shredded

  1/3 cup unsweetened almond milk

  2 tablespoons unsalted butter, melted

  2 large organic eggs, beaten

DIRECTIONS :

1. Preheat a mini waffle iron and then grease it.
2. In a large bowl, place flax seeds meal, flour, protein powder, baking powder, and mix well.
3. Stir in the Cheddar cheese.
4. Introduce to a medium bowl, all ingredients and mix until well combined.
5. Add the egg mixture into the bowl with flax seeds meal mixture and mix until well combined.

6. Place desired amount of the mixture into preheated waffle iron and cook for about 4-5 minutes or until golden brown.
7. Repeat with the remaining mixture.
8. Serve warm.

NUTRITION : Calories: 187Net Carb: 1.8gFat: 14.5gSaturated Fat: 5gCarbohydrates: 4.Dietary Fiber: 3.1g Sugar: 0.4gProtein: 8g

Chicken & Ham Chaffles

Preparation time : 10 minutes

Cooking Time : 16 Minutes

Servings : 2

INGREDIENTS :

   ¼ cup grass-fed cooked chicken, chopped

   1 ounce sugar-free ham, chopped

   1 organic egg, beaten

   ¼ cup Swiss cheese, shredded

   ¼ cup Mozzarella cheese, shredded

DIRECTIONS :

1. Preheat a mini waffle iron and then grease it.
2. Introduce to a medium bowl, all ingredients and mix until well combined.
3. Place ¼ of the mixture into preheated waffle iron and cook for about 4 minutes or until golden brown.
4. Repeat with the remaining mixture.
5. Serve warm.

NUTRITION : Calories: 71Net Carb: 0.7gFat: 4.2gSaturated Fat: 2gCarbohydrates: 0.8gDietary Fiber: 0.1g Sugar: 0.2gProtein: 7.4g

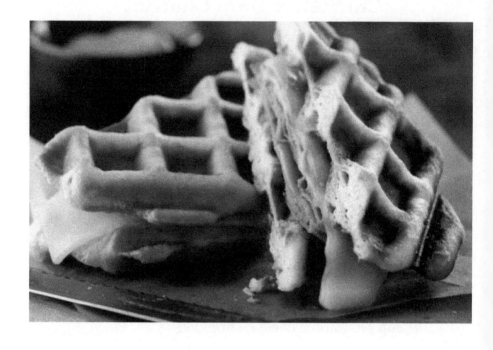

Herb Chaffles

Preparation time : 10 minutes

Cooking Time : 12 Minutes

Servings : 2

INGREDIENTS :

    4 tablespoons almond flour

    1 tablespoon coconut flour

    1 teaspoon mixed dried herbs

    ½ teaspoon organic baking powder

    ¼ teaspoon garlic powder

    ¼ teaspoon onion powder

    Salt and ground black pepper, to taste

    ¼ cup cream cheese, softened

    3 large organic eggs

    ½ cup cheddar cheese, grated

    1/3 cup Parmesan cheese, grated

DIRECTIONS :

1. Preheat a waffle iron and then grease it.
2. In a bowl, mix the flours, dried herbs, baking powder, seasoning, and mix well.
3. In a separate bowl, put cream cheese and eggs and beat until well combined.

4. Add the flour mixture, cheddar, and Parmesan cheese, and mix until well combined.

5. Place the desired amount of the mixture into preheated waffle iron and cook for about 2–3 minutes.

6. Repeat with the remaining mixture.

7. Serve warm.

NUTRITION : Calories 240 Net Carb: g Total Fat 19 g Saturated Fat 5 gCholesterol 176 mgSodium 280 mg Total Carbs 4 gFiber 1.6 g Sugar 0.7 gProtein 12.3 g

Scallion Chaffles

Preparation time : 6 minutes

Cooking Time : 8 Minutes

Servings : 2

INGREDIENTS :

1 organic egg, beaten

½ cup Mozzarella cheese, shredded

1 tablespoon scallion, chopped

½ teaspoon Italian seasoning

DIRECTIONS :

1. Preheat a mini waffle iron and then grease it.

2. Introduce to a medium bowl, all ingredients and mix until well combined

3. Put a portion of the mixture in the preheated waffle iron and cook until golden brown, or around 4 minutes.

4. Repeat with the mixture that remains.

5. Serve it hot.

NUTRITION : Calories: 5et Carb: 0.7gFat: 3.8gSaturated Fat: 1.5gCarbohydrates: 0.8gDietary Fiber: 0.g Sugar: 0.3gProtein: 4.8g

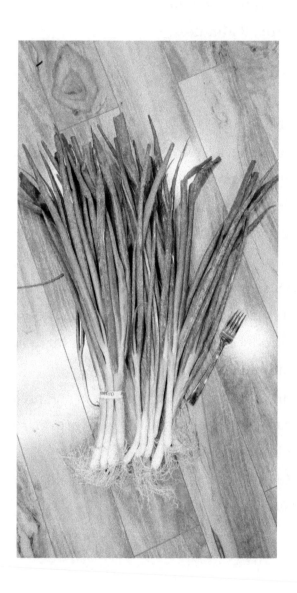

Eggs Benedict Chaffle

Preparation time : 6 minutes

Cooking Time : 10 Minutes

Servings : 2

INGREDIENTS :

> For the chaffle:
>
> 2 egg whites
>
> 2 Tbsp almond flour
>
> 1 Tbsp sour cream
>
> ½ cup mozzarella cheese
>
> For the hollandaise:
>
> ½ cup salted butter
>
> 4 egg yolks
>
> 2 Tbsp lemon juice
>
> For the poached eggs:
>
> 2 eggs
>
> 1 Tbsp white vinegar
>
> 3 oz deli ham

DIRECTIONS :

1. Whip egg white until frothy, then mix in remaining **INGREDIENTS** .
2. Turn on the waffle maker to heat and oil it with cooking spray.
3. Cook for 7 minutes until golden brown.
4. Remove shuffle and repeat with remaining batter.
5. Fill half the pot with water and bring to a boil.
6. Place a heat-safe bowl on top of the pot, ensuring the bottom doesn't touch the boiling water.
7. Heat butter to boiling in a microwave.
8. Add yolks to a double boiler bowl and bring to a boil.
9. Add hot butter to the bowl and whisk briskly. Cook until the egg yolk mixture has thickened.
10. Remove bowl from pot and add in lemon juice. Set aside.
11. Add more water to the pot if needed to make the poached eggs (water should completely cover the eggs). Bring to a simmer. Add white vinegar to water.
12. Break eggs into boiling water and cook for 1 minute 30 seconds. Remove using a slotted spoon.
13. Warm waffles in the toaster for 2-3 minutes. Top with ham, poached eggs, and hollandaise sauce.

NUTRITION :Carbs: 4 g;Fat: 26 g;Protein: 26 g;Calories: 365

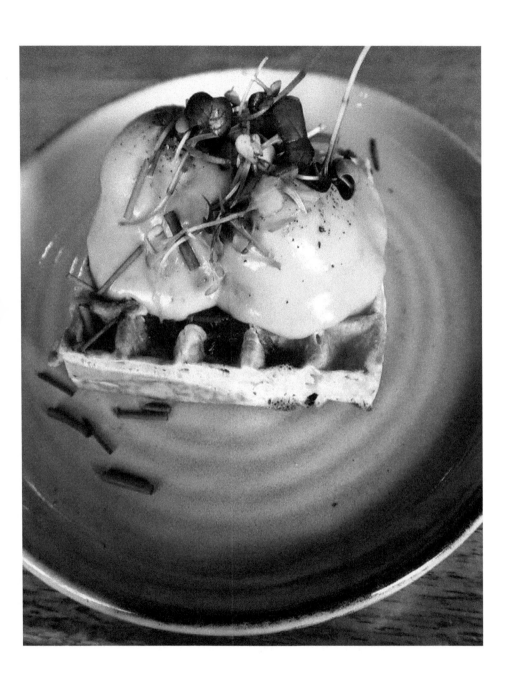

Chicken Bacon Chaffle

Preparation time : 6 minutes

Cooking Time : 5 Minutes

Servings : 2

INGREDIENTS :

    1 egg

    ⅓ cup cooked chicken, diced

    1 piece of bacon, cooked and crumbled

    ⅓ cup shredded cheddar jack cheese

    1 tsp powdered ranch dressing

DIRECTIONS :

1. Turn on the waffle maker to heat and oil it with cooking spray.
2. Mix egg, dressing, and Monterey cheese in a small bowl.
3. Add bacon and chicken.
4. Introduce half of the batter to the waffle maker and cook for 3-minutes.
5. Remove and cook remaining batter to make a second chaffle.
6. Let chaffles sit for 2 minutes before serving.

NUTRITION :Carbs: 2 g;Fat: 14 g;Protein: 16 g;Calories: 200

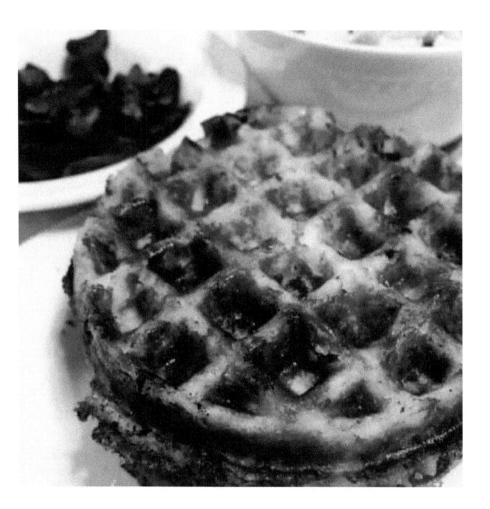

Bacon & Veggies Chaffles

Servings : 6

Cooking Time : 24 Minutes

INGREDIENTS :

   2 cooked bacon slices, crumbled

   ½ cup frozen chopped spinach, thawed and squeezed

   ½ cup cauliflower rice

   2 organic eggs

   ½ cup Cheddar cheese, shredded

   ½ cup Mozzarella cheese, shredded

   ¼ cup Parmesan cheese, grated

   1 tablespoon butter, melted

   1 teaspoon garlic powder

   1 teaspoon onion powder

DIRECTIONS :

1. Preheat a mini waffle iron and then grease it.
2. Introduce to a medium bowl, all ingredients and mix until well combined In a bowl
3. Fold in the blueberries.
4. Divide the mixture into 6 portions.
5. Place 1 portion of the mixture into preheated waffle iron and cook for about 3-4 minutes or until golden brown.

6. Repeat with the remaining mixture.

7. Serve warm.

NUTRITION : Calories: 10et Carb: 1.2gFat: 8.4gSaturated Fat: 4.6gCarbohydrates: 1.5gDietary Fiber: 0.3g Sugar: 0.6gProtein: 7.1g

Garlic Cheese Chaffle Bread Sticks

Servings : 8

Cooking Time : 5 Minutes

INGREDIENTS :

> 1 medium egg
>
> ½ cup mozzarella cheese, grated
>
> 2 Tbsp almond flour
>
> ½ tsp garlic powder
>
> ½ tsp oregano
>
> ½ tsp salt
>
> For the toppings:
>
> 2 Tbsp butter, unsalted softened
>
> ½ tsp garlic powder
>
> ¼ cup grated mozzarella cheese
>
> 2 tsp dried oregano for sprinkling

DIRECTIONS :

1. Turn on the waffle maker to heat and oil it with cooking spray.
2. Beat egg in a bowl.
3. Add mozzarella, garlic powder, flour, oregano, and salt, and mix.
4. With a spoon put a portion of the batter into the waffle maker.

5. Close and cook for minutes. Remove cooked chaffle.

6. Repeat with remaining batter.

7. Place chaffles on a tray and preheat the grill.

8. Mix butter with garlic powder and spread over the chaffles.

9. Sprinkle mozzarella over top and cook under the broiler for 2-3 minutes, until cheese has melted.

NUTRITION :Carbs: 1 g;Fat: 7 g;Protein: 4 g;Calories: 74

Simple Savory Waffles

Preparation time : 6 minutes

Cooking Time : 8 Minutes

Servings : 4

INGREDIENTS :

    1 large organic egg, beaten

    ½ cup Cheddar cheese, shredded

    Pinch of salt

    freshly ground black pepper

DIRECTIONS :

1. Preheat a mini waffle iron and then grease it.
2. Introduce to a medium bowl, all ingredients and mix until well combined
3. Put a portion of the mixture in the preheated waffle iron and cook until golden brown, or around 4 minutes.
4. Repeat with the mixture that remains.
5. Serve it hot..

NUTRITION : Calories: 150Net Carb: 0.Fat: 11.9gSaturated Fat: 6.7gCarbohydrates: 0.6gDietary Fiber: 0g Sugar: 0.3gProtein: 10.2g

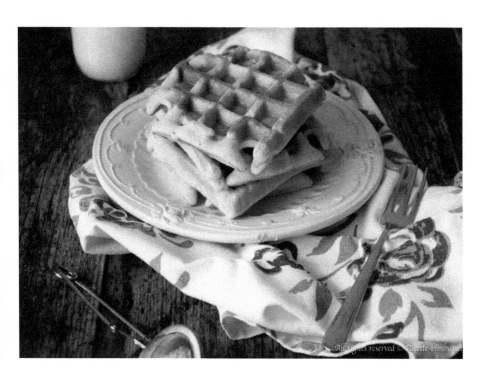

Parmesan Garlic Chaffle

Preparation time : 6 minutes

Cooking Time : 5 Minutes

Servings : 2

INGREDIENTS :

    1 Tbsp fresh garlic minced

    2 Tbsp butter

    1-oz cream cheese, cubed

    2 Tbsp almond flour

    1 tsp baking soda

    2 large eggs

    1 tsp dried chives

    ½ cup parmesan cheese, shredded

    ¾ cup mozzarella cheese, shredded

DIRECTIONS :

1. Heat cream cheese and butter in a saucepan over medium-low until melted.
2. Add garlic and cook, stirring, for minutes.
3. Turn on the waffle maker to heat and oil it with cooking spray.
4. In a small mixing bowl, whisk together flour and baking soda, then set aside.

77

5. In a separate bowl, beat eggs for 1 minute 30 seconds on high, then add in cream cheese mixture and beat for 60 seconds more.
6. Add flour mixture, chives, and cheeses to the bowl and stir well.
7. Add ¼ cup batter to the waffle maker.
8. Close and cook for 4 minutes, until golden brown.
9. Repeat for remaining batter.
10. Add favorite toppings and serve.

NUTRITION :Carbs: 5 g;Fat: 33 g;Protein: 19 g;Calories: 38 5

Chicken & Veggies Chaffles

Preparation time : 10 minutes

Cooking Time : 15 Minutes

Servings : 2

INGREDIENTS :

      1/3 cup cooked grass-fed chicken, chopped

      1/3 cup cooked spinach, chopped

      1/3 cup marinated artichokes, chopped

      1 organic egg, beaten

      1/3 cup Mozzarella cheese, shredded

      1 ounce cream cheese, softened

      ¼ teaspoon garlic powder

DIRECTIONS :

1. Preheat a mini waffle iron and then grease it.
2. Introduce to a medium bowl, all ingredients and mix until well combined.
3. Place 1/of the mixture into preheated waffle iron and cook for about 4-5 minutes or until golden brown.
4. Repeat with the remaining mixture.
5. Serve warm.

NUTRITION : Calories: 95Net Carb: 1.3gFat: 5.8gSaturated Fat: 1.3gCarbohydrates: 2.2gDietary Fiber: 0.9g Sugar: 0.3gProtein: 8.

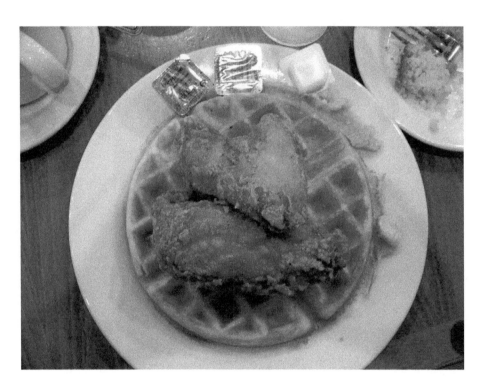

Turkey Chaffles

Preparation time : 10 minutes

Cooking Time : 16 Minutes

Servings : 2

INGREDIENTS :

    ½ cup cooked turkey meat, chopped

    2 organic eggs, beaten

    ½ cup Parmesan cheese, grated

    ½ cup Mozzarella, shredded

    ¼ teaspoon poultry seasoning

    ¼ teaspoon onion powder

DIRECTIONS :

1. Preheat a mini waffle iron and then grease it.
2. Introduce to a medium bowl, all ingredients and mix until well combined.
3. Place ¼ of the mixture into preheated waffle iron and cook for about 4 minutes or until golden brown.
4. Repeat with the remaining mixture.
5. Serve warm.

NUTRITION : Calories: 108Net Carb: 0.5gFat: 1gSaturated Fat: 2.6gCarbohydrates: 0.5gDietary Fiber: 0g Sugar: 0.2gProtein: 12.9 g

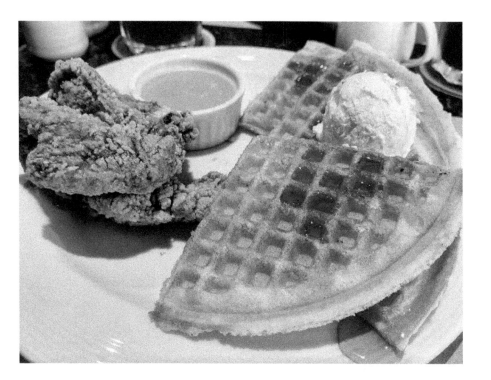

Chicken & Zucchini Chaffles

Servings : 9

Cooking Time : 0 Minutes

INGREDIENTS :

    4 ounces cooked grass-fed chicken, chopped

    2 cups zucchini, shredded and squeezed

    ¼ cup scallion, chopped

    2 large organic eggs

    ½ cup Mozzarella cheese, shredded

    ½ cup Cheddar cheese, shredded

    ½ cup blanched almond flour

    1 teaspoon organic baking powder

    ½ teaspoon garlic salt

    ½ teaspoon onion powder

DIRECTIONS :

1. Preheat a waffle iron and then grease it.
2. Introduce to a medium bowl, all ingredients and mix until well combined.
3. Divide the mixture into 9 portions.
4. Place 1 portion of the mixture into preheated waffle iron and cook for about 2-3 minutes or until golden brown.
5. Repeat with the remaining mixture.

6. Serve warm.

NUTRITION : Calories: 108Net Carb: 2gFat: 6.9gSaturated Fat: 2.2gCarbohydrates: 3.1gDietary Fiber: 1.1g Sugar: 0.Protein: 8.8g

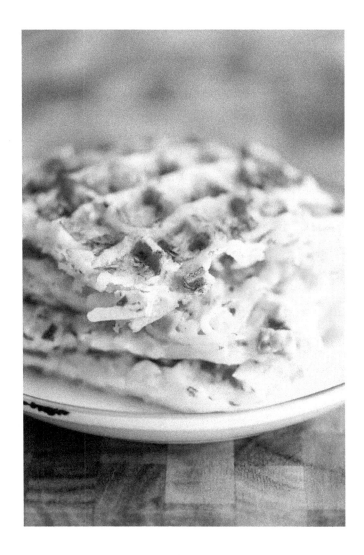

Pepperoni Chaffles

Preparation time : 5 minutes

Cooking Time : 5 Minutes

Servings : 2

INGREDIENTS :

    1 organic egg, beaten

    ½ cup Mozzarella cheese, shredded

    2 tablespoons turkey pepperoni slice, chopped

    1 tablespoon sugar-free pizza sauce

    ¼ teaspoon Italian seasoning

DIRECTIONS :

1. Preheat a waffle iron and then grease it.
2. Introduce in a bowl, all the ingredients and mix well.
3. Place the mixture into preheated waffle iron and cook for about 5 minutes or until golden brown.
4. Serve warm.

NUTRITION : Calories: 119Net Carb: 2.4gFat: 7.gSaturated Fat: 3gCarbohydrates: 2.7gDietary Fiber: 0.3g Sugar: 0.9gProtein: 10.3g

Hot Sauce Jalapeño Chaffles

Preparation time : 6 minutes

Cooking Time : 8 Minutes

Servings : 2

INGREDIENTS :

 ½ cup plus 2 teaspoons Cheddar cheese, shredded and divided

 1 organic egg, beaten

 6 jalapeño pepper slices

 ¼ teaspoon hot sauce

 Pinch of salt

DIRECTIONS :

1. Preheat a mini waffle iron and then grease it.
2. In a bowl, place ½ cup of cheese and remaining ingredients and mix until well combined.
3. Place about 1 teaspoon of cheese in the bottom of the waffle maker for about seconds before adding the mixture.
4. Introduce a portion of the mixture into preheated waffle iron and cook for about 3-minutes or until golden brown.
5. Repeat with the remaining cheese and mixture.

6. Serve warm.

NUTRITION : Calories: 153Net Carb: 0.6gFat: 12.2gSaturated Fat: Carbohydrates: 0.7gDietary Fiber: 0.1g Sugar: 0.4gProtein: 10.3g

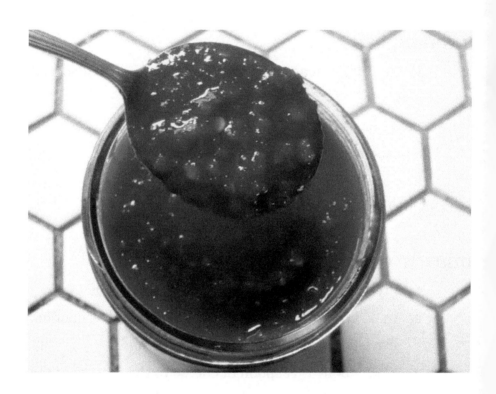

Chicken Chaffles

Preparation time : 10 minutes

Cooking Time : 15 Minutes

Servings : 2

INGREDIENTS :

2 oz chicken breasts, cooked, shredded

1/2 cup mozzarella cheese, finely shredded

2 eggs

6 tbsp parmesan cheese, finely shredded

1 cup zucchini, grated

½ cup almond flour

1tsp baking powder

¼ tsp garlic powder

¼ tsp black pepper, ground

½ tsp Italian seasoning

¼ tsp salt

DIRECTIONS :

1. Put a pinch of salt on the zucchini and set it aside for a few minutes. Squeeze out the excess water.
2. Warm up your mini waffle maker.
3. Mix chicken, almond flour, baking powder, cheeses, garlic powder, salt, pepper and seasonings in a bowl.

4. Use another small bow for beating eggs. Add them to squeezed zucchini, mix well.

5. Combine the chicken and egg mixture, and mix.

6. For a crispy crust, add a teaspoon of shredded cheese to the waffle maker and cook for 30 seconds.

7. Then, pour the mixture into the waffle maker and cook for 5 minutes or until crispy.

8. Carefully remove. Repeat with remaining batter the same steps.

9. Enjoy!

NUTRITION : Calories 35Kcal Fats: 5g Carbs: 3g Protein: 11g

Garlicky Chicken Chaffles

Preparation time : 6 minutes

Cooking Time : 12 Minutes

Servings : 2

INGREDIENTS :

      1 organic egg, beaten

      1/3 cup grass-fed cooked chicken, chopped

      1/3 cup Mozzarella cheese, shredded

      ¼ teaspoon garlic, minced

      ¼ teaspoon dried basil, crushed

DIRECTIONS :

1. Preheat a mini waffle iron and then grease it.
2. Introduce all ingredients in a medium bowl and, with a fork, mix until well mixed.
3. Put a portion of the mixture in the preheated waffle iron and cook until golden brown, or around 4-6 minutes.
4. 4. Repeat with the mixture that remains.
5. Serve it hot.

NUTRITION : Calories: 81Net Carb: 0.5gFat: 3.7gSaturated Fat: 1.4gCarbohydrates: 0.5gDietary Fiber: 0g Sugar: 0.2gProtein: 10.9g

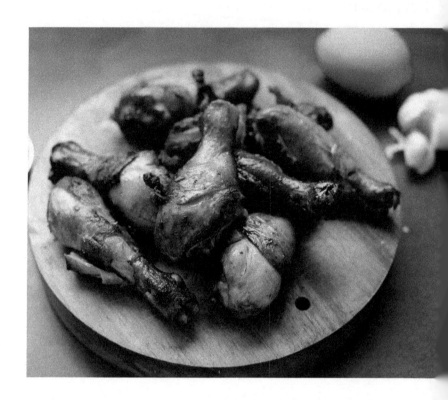

Garlic Herb Blend Seasoning Chaffles

Preparation time : 6 minutes

Cooking Time : 8 Minutes

Servings : 2

INGREDIENTS :

　　1 large organic egg, beaten

　　¼ cup Parmesan cheese, shredded

　　¼ cup Mozzarella cheese, shredded

　　½ tablespoon butter, melted

　　1 teaspoon garlic herb blend seasoning

　　Salt, to taste

DIRECTIONS :

1. Preheat a mini waffle iron and then grease it.
2. Introduce all ingredients toa medium bowl and, with a fork, mix until well mixed.
3. Put a portion of the mixture in the preheated waffle iron and cook until golden brown, or around 4 minutes.
4. Repeat with the mixture that remains.
5. Serve it hot.

NUTRITION : Calories: 115Net Carb: 1.1gFat: 8.8gSaturated Fat: 4.7gCarbohydrates: 1.2gDietary Fiber: 0.1g Sugar: 0.2gProtein: 8g

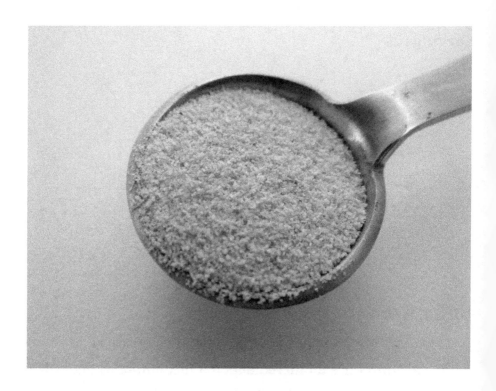

Protein Cheddar Chaffles

Servings : 8

Cooking Time : 48 Minutes

INGREDIENTS :

½ cup golden flax seeds meal

½ cup almond flour

2 tablespoons unflavored whey protein powder

1 teaspoon organic baking powder

Salt and ground black pepper, to taste

¾ cup cheddar cheese, shredded

1/3 cup unsweetened almond milk

2 tablespoons unsalted butter, melted

2 large organic eggs, beaten

DIRECTIONS :

1. Preheat a mini waffle iron and then grease it.
2. In a large bowl, add flax seeds meal, flour, protein powder, baking powder, and mix well.
3. Stir in the cheddar cheese.
4. In another bowl, add the remaining **INGREDIENTS** and beat until well combined.
5. Add the egg mixture into the bowl with flax seeds meal mixture and mix until well combined.

6. Place desired amount of the mixture into preheated waffle iron.
7. Cook for about 4–6 minutes.
8. Repeat with the remaining mixture.
9. Serve warm.

NUTRITION : Calories 187 Net Carbs 1.8 g Total Fat 14.5 g Saturated Fat 5 gCholesterol 65 mgSodium 134 mg Total Carbs 4.9 gFiber 3.1 g Sugar 0.4 gProtein 8 g

Garlic & Onion Powder Chaffles

Preparation time : 5 minutes

Cooking Time : 5 Minutes

Servings : 2

INGREDIENTS :

>1 organic egg, beaten
>
>¼ cup Cheddar cheese, shredded
>
>2 tablespoons almond flour
>
>½ teaspoon organic baking powder
>
>¼ teaspoon garlic powder
>
>¼ teaspoon onion powder
>
>Pinch of salt

DIRECTIONS :

1. Preheat a waffle iron and then grease it.
2. In a bowl, introduce all ingredients and beat until well combined.
3. Place the mixture into preheated waffle iron and cook for about 5 minutes or until golden brown.
4. Serve warm.

NUTRITION : Calories: 274Net Carb: 3.3gFat: 21.3gSaturated Fat: 7.8gCarbohydrates: Dietary Fiber: 1.7g Sugar: 1.4gProtein: 12.8g

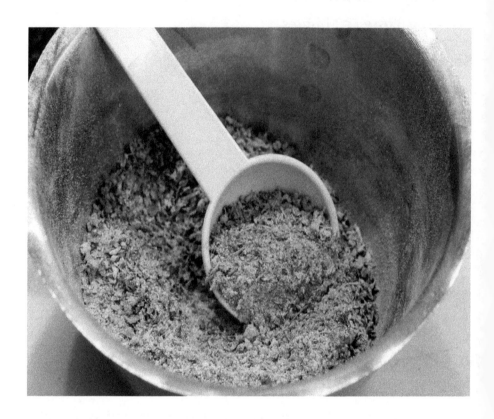

Savory Bagel Seasoning Chaffles

Servings :4

Cooking Time : 5 Minutes

INGREDIENTS :

2 tbsps. everything bagel seasoning

2 eggs

1 cup mozzarella cheese

1/2 cup grated parmesan

DIRECTIONS :

1. Preheat the square waffle maker and grease with cooking spray.

2. Mix eggs, mozzarella cheese and grated cheese in a bowl.

3. Introduce half of the batter in the waffle maker.

4. Sprinkle 1 tbsp. of the everything bagel seasoning over batter.

5. Cover.

6. Cook chaffles for about 3-4 minutes Utes.

7. Repeat with the remaining batter.

8. Serve hot and enjoy!

NUTRITION : Protein: 71kcal Fat: 125kcal Carbohydrates: 13kcal

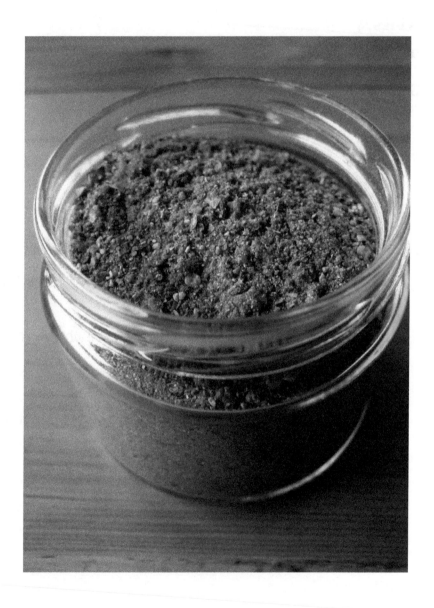

Dried Herbs Chaffles

Preparation time : 6 minutes

Cooking Time : 8 Minutes

Servings : 2

INGREDIENTS :

     1 organic egg, beaten

     ½ cup Cheddar cheese, shredded

     1 tablespoon almond flour

     Pinch of dried thyme, crushed

     Pinch of dried rosemary, crushed

DIRECTIONS :

1. Preheat a mini waffle iron and then grease it.
2. In a bowl, place all the ingredients and beat thoroughly.
3. Put a portion of the mixture into preheated waffle iron and cook for about 4 minutes or until golden brown.
4. Repeat with the remaining mixture.
5. Serve warm.

NUTRITION : Calories: 1Net Carb: 0.9gFat: 13.4gSaturated Fat: 6.8gCarbohydrates: 1.3gDietary Fiber: 0.4g Sugar: 0.4gProtein: 9.8g

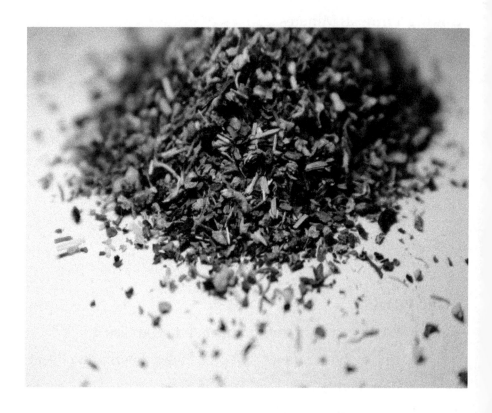

Sour Cream Protein Chaffles

Preparation time : 10 minutes

Cooking Time : 16 Minutes

Servings : 2

INGREDIENTS :

6 organic eggs

½ cup sour cream

½ cup unsweetened whey protein powder

1 teaspoon organic baking powder

½ teaspoon salt

1 cup Cheddar cheese, shredded

DIRECTIONS :

1. Preheat a waffle iron and then grease it.
2. In a medium bowl, introduce all ingredients and mix until well combined.
3. Place ¼ of the mixture into preheated waffle iron and cook for about 4 minutes or until golden brown.
4. Repeat with the remaining mixture.
5. Serve warm.
6.

NUTRITION : Calories: 324Net Carb: 3.Fat: 22.6gSaturated Fat: 11.9gCarbohydrates: 3.6gDietary Fiber: 0g Sugar: 1.3gProtein: 27.3g

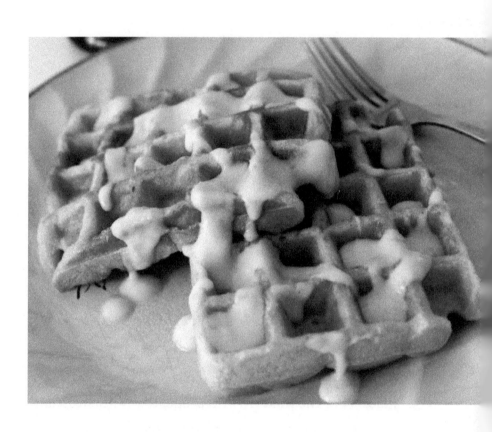

Zucchini & Basil Chaffles

Preparation time : 6 minutes

Cooking Time : 10 Minutes

Servings : 2

INGREDIENTS :

    1 organic egg, beaten

    ¼ cup Mozzarella cheese, shredded

    2 tablespoons Parmesan cheese, grated

    ½ of small zucchini, grated and squeezed

    ¼ teaspoon dried basil, crushed

    Freshly ground black pepper, as required

DIRECTIONS :

1. Preheat a mini waffle iron and then grease it.
2. Introduce all ingredients in a medium bowl and, with a fork, mix until well mixed.
3. Put a portion of the mixture in the preheated waffle iron and cook until golden brown, or around 4 minutes.
4. Repeat with the mixture that remains.
5. Serve it hot.

NUTRITION : Calories: Net Carb: 1gFat: 4.1gSaturated Fat: 1.7gCarbohydrates: 1.3gDietary Fiber: 0.3g Sugar: 0.7gProtein: 6.1g

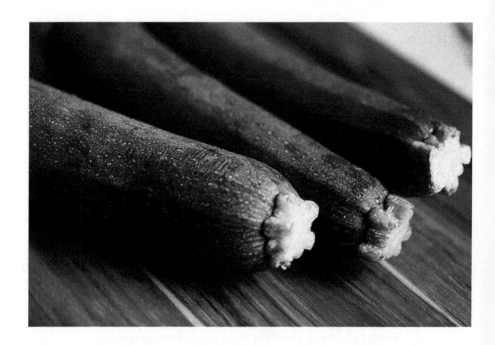